CONTENTS

Introduction 4

Chapter 1: Introduction to Your Postpartum Body 7

Chapter 2: Nutrition for Recovery, Not Just Weight Loss ... 14

Chapter 3: Gentle Exercises for Body and Mind 20

Chapter 4: Battling Fatigue: Sleep and Energy 27

Chapter 5: Realistic Fitness Plans for Busy Mums 34

Chapter 6: Postpartum Mental Health: Nurturing the Mind and Spirit ... 41

Chapter 7: Rediscovering Your Identity After Baby 49

Chapter 8: Busting the Bounce-Back Myth 55

Chapter 9: Advanced Postpartum Fitness: Building Strength When You're Ready ... 61

Chapter 10: How to Build Long-Term Sustainable Habits ... 70

Conclusion: You've Got This, Mum 76

About The Author 80

Mum's Back: The Honest Guide to Post-Pregnancy Weight Loss, Fitness, and Mental Health.

The Practical Path to Regaining Strength, Energy, and Confidence After Baby

Lauren Nikora

© Copyright 2024 - All rights reserved.

INTRODUCTION

Welcome to the postpartum rollercoaster. Whether you're a first-time mum or adding another little one to your growing tribe, this journey is both wonderful and, let's be honest, a bit overwhelming. If you're sitting there, sleep-deprived, wondering when you'll start feeling like yourself again, don't worry—you're not alone. And no, the answer isn't "by next Tuesday." Recovery is a slow dance, not a race.

This book is here to help you through that delicate transition—from feeling like your body isn't quite your own, to reclaiming your strength, energy, and confidence. Let's be real: this isn't about some magical "snap back" to your pre-baby self. You've spent the better part of a year creating a human, and that deserves a bit more credit than trying to fit back into your old jeans by next month.

We're focusing on real, practical steps that fit into the chaos of motherhood—no crash diets, no intense fitness regimes, and definitely no guilt. You've got enough on your plate without adding unrealistic expectations of bouncing back as if the past nine months never happened. This book is about progress, not perfection. It's about you, moving at your own pace, rebuilding the healthiest, happiest version of yourself one step at a time.

◆ ◆ ◆

What to Expect from This Book:

In these pages, you'll find simple, practical advice for regaining your strength, energy, and mental wellbeing. We're not going to overwhelm you with intense schedules or fancy jargon—because let's face it, who's got time for that? Instead, I'm giving you a toolkit for the postpartum journey that's adaptable and easy to fit into real life.

You'll get step-by-step guides on:

- *Understanding what's happening to your postpartum body (spoiler: it's not supposed to bounce back overnight, and anyone who tells you otherwise can jog on).*
- *Eating well without diving into restrictive diets or giving up the food that keeps you sane (yes, that means chocolate and a cuppa are still on the menu).*
- *Gentle exercises that fit around your schedule and help you rebuild strength—without demanding hours of time you don't have.*
- *Navigating the emotional side of motherhood, because it's not just about your body—your mental health is just as important.*

You'll learn how to make small changes that lead to lasting results, and how to avoid the common traps new mums often fall into when they're trying to "get back" to normal. Spoiler alert: the normal you're heading for isn't the same as the old normal. And that's okay. In fact, it's more than okay—it's pretty fantastic.

Progress, Not Perfection

If you're looking for a quick fix or a magic formula to make everything go back to the way it was, this isn't the book for you. But if you want honest advice, realistic goals, and a bit of a laugh along the way, you're in the right place. We'll talk about everything from body changes to meal prepping, with a good dose of reassurance that you're doing brilliantly—even when it doesn't feel like it.

And here's the golden rule to keep in mind: be kind to yourself. You've done something incredible, and your body deserves patience and love, not punishment. This book is your guide to navigating postpartum recovery with grace, humour, and a focus on feeling good in the long run—not just in the short term.

So, shall we get started? Grab a cuppa, put your feet up (if you can), and let's take this journey together, one small step at a time. You've got this, and I'm here to remind you that even on the tough days, you're already doing an amazing job.

CHAPTER 1: INTRODUCTION TO YOUR POSTPARTUM BODY

Welcome to the aftermath, love. You've been through a physical marathon, and now that the main event is over, it's time to get familiar with the landscape of your new body. Don't worry, you're in good company—whether it's your first time or you're adding to the brood, the body you've lived in for the last nine months is still yours, it's just... different. It's a bit like waking up after a wild party (except you've been the host, guest, and entertainment all rolled into one). This chapter will be your guide to what's happening inside that brilliant body of yours. Spoiler: it's all normal, even if it feels like someone's hit shuffle on everything.

◆ ◆ ◆

Hormonal Havoc – The Not-So-Fun Disco Inside Your Body

So, you made it through the pregnancy rollercoaster, but those hormones aren't quite ready to let you off the ride just yet. During pregnancy, your body's oestrogen and progesterone levels shot up higher than your cravings for late-night chippy runs. But now, those hormones have decided to stage a dramatic exit. This dip in hormones can leave you feeling deflated, both emotionally and physically—literally like a balloon losing its air, and figuratively when it comes to mood swings.

What To Expect With Hormonal Changes:

- ***Mood Swings:*** *One minute you're tearing up at a nappy advert, the next you're shouting at the toaster for burning your bread. It's okay—you're not losing it, it's just your hormones taking their sweet time to recalibrate.*

- ***Hair Loss (Sorry, It's Not Over Yet):*** *During pregnancy, your hair probably felt thicker and shinier than ever. But postpartum, it's common to shed that extra hair. Don't panic—it will grow back, but it's a bit like autumn for your scalp right now.*

- ***Energy Slumps:*** *Between the hormonal shifts and sleep deprivation, your energy might feel like it's been stolen by a toddler who's also hiding your car keys. It's* frustrating, but normal.

How To Help Your Hormonal Balance:

1. ***Eat Hormone-Friendly Foods****: Balance your meals with healthy fats (think avocados, nuts, seeds) that help with hormonal regulation. They're a much better choice than the chocolate stash calling your name at 2 a.m.*

2. ***Sleep (If You Can)****: Easier said than done, right? But try to sneak in naps when you can because sleep helps regulate cortisol (the stress hormone). And no, that doesn't mean trying to sleep when the baby sleeps—unless, of course, you can manage it without obsessively checking if they're breathing.*

3. ***Don't Rush to 'Fix' Yourself****: Your body is still healing. Give it time, and don't expect to feel 'normal' right away. Spoiler alert: 'normal' might look a bit different now, and that's*

okay.

◆ ◆ ◆

Why Your Metabolism Feels Like It's Gone on Holiday

You might have heard people say breastfeeding is a magic trick for weight loss. While it's true that breastfeeding burns extra calories (roughly 300-500 per day), it doesn't work the same for everyone. Your body is also holding onto reserves, making sure it can keep up with milk production. Add to this the fact that your metabolism often slows down postpartum as your body adjusts to life post-baby, and it's no wonder you're not feeling like running a marathon just yet.

What's Happening With Your Metabolism:

- *Recovery Mode: Your body has gone through labour and delivery, which means it's in recovery. Your metabolic rate naturally slows during this time.*
- *Energy Conservation: If you're sleep-deprived (and let's be honest, who isn't?), your body might hold onto fat because it's in conservation mode, storing energy for all those midnight feedings.*

How To Boost Your Metabolism (Gently):

1. *Start Moving (Slowly): Gentle movement, like walking or light stretching, can help boost your metabolism without overloading your body. No need for a hard-core workout— just strolling with the pram is a great way to get things going.*
2. *Snack Smart: If you're feeling ravenous between meals, don't reach for sugary snacks. Instead, opt for something*

with protein and fibre, like hummus with veg sticks, or an apple with peanut butter. These keep your energy stable and metabolism ticking along.

3. **Stay Hydrated**: *This sounds simple, but keeping your hydration levels up is key to helping digestion and energy production. Drink water throughout the day, and herbal teas if you want to feel a bit fancy.*

◆ ◆ ◆

Diastasis Recti: What It Is and What It Isn't

Here's the fun bit: diastasis recti. If you've noticed a gap down the middle of your tummy, that's because your abdominal muscles have stretched apart to make space for your little one. Don't worry—it's completely normal. But doing crunches to get your old belly back? Please, no. That's only going to make it worse.

What Diastasis Recti Is:

- *A natural separation of your abdominal muscles. It happens to most women during pregnancy as your uterus expands.*
- *It can cause your stomach to look more pronounced (even months after giving birth), but it's nothing you've done wrong.*

How To Help Heal Diastasis Recti:

1. **Pelvic Floor Exercises**: *Kegels are your best friend now. They strengthen the muscles that support your bladder, uterus, and bowels. You can do them anywhere—while feeding the baby, standing in a queue, or lying down in bed.*
2. **Gentle Core Work**: *Think about gentle core exercises like pelvic tilts or breathing exercises that engage the deep core muscles without straining the gap.*

3. ***Avoid Crunches and Sit-ups****: These will do more harm than good if you've got diastasis recti. Stick to low-impact exercises until your muscles heal.*

The Myth of the "Snap Back"

Here's the truth: there is no 'snap back'. Those celebrities who seem to magically shrink down days after giving birth? Well, they've got nannies, personal chefs, trainers, and a lot more going on behind the scenes than you do. You, on the other hand, are juggling a baby, housework, and life on very little sleep. So, don't buy into the pressure of "snapping back." You've just done something miraculous—growing and birthing a human—and your body deserves more than a race to fit back into pre-pregnancy jeans.

Forget The Snap Back—Focus On Feeling Good Instead:

1. ***Set Realistic Goals****: Instead of focusing on weight loss, think about what will make you feel good—whether that's having more energy, finding a new daily rhythm, or just fitting in some 'me time.'*
2. ***Be Kind to Yourself****: Comparison is the thief of joy, so stop comparing yourself to anyone else—especially to Insta-mums with their post-baby body shots. Your body is unique, and so is your journey.*
3. ***Celebrate the Wins****: Whether it's getting through the day without stepping on a toy or managing a short walk, celebrate the small victories.*

Breastfeeding and Weight Loss: A Reality Check

You've probably heard that breastfeeding can help shed the baby weight. It's true, breastfeeding can burn extra calories, but it's not a magic cure. For some mums, breastfeeding makes weight loss trickier because the body holds onto extra reserves to keep up milk production. And that's perfectly okay.

What You Should Know About Breastfeeding And Weight:

- *Calorie Burn*: Yes, breastfeeding burns calories, but not enough to warrant a drastic transformation.
- *Hormonal Hold-Up*: The hormones involved in milk production can also cause your body to hold onto fat—your body's way of making sure it has enough fuel to feed the baby.

How To Keep Things In Perspective:

1. *Focus on Nourishment*: Prioritise eating nourishing meals that support both you and your baby's health over worrying about fitting into your old clothes.
2. *Be Patient with Your Body*: It took nine months to grow a baby, so give yourself at least that much time to heal and recover.

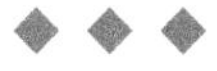

Patience, Progress, and Kindness

So, what's the takeaway here? Give yourself grace. Your body has done something extraordinary, and it deserves time to heal and rebuild. This is about patience, progress, and kindness—not perfection. Each step forward is a victory, no matter how small.

Remember, this journey isn't about getting back to who you were —it's about embracing the strong, resilient woman you are now. One day at a time.

CHAPTER 2: NUTRITION FOR RECOVERY, NOT JUST WEIGHT LOSS

Alright, love, it's time to talk about food—arguably one of the most comforting and complicated topics postpartum. You've spent nine months making room for cravings and indulging in foods that kept you going. Now, as you embark on your recovery journey, we're shifting the focus. But don't worry, this isn't going to be a lecture on cutting out the foods you love or existing solely on carrot sticks and kale.

This chapter is all about nourishing your body as it heals. You've done the hard work of growing a human, so now it's about feeding yourself in a way that restores your energy, supports your mood, and yes, gently helps with weight loss—but at your own pace.

Understanding What Your Body Really Needs

Your body has been through the equivalent of a marathon. It's exhausted, depleted, and in need of some serious TLC. What it doesn't need is a crash diet or some kind of punishment for gaining weight during pregnancy. Postpartum is about repair and recovery first, and weight loss second.

Let's break it down. To fuel your body properly, you need to focus on three key nutrients: **protein, fibre**, and **healthy fats**. These are the essentials that help rebuild muscle, regulate digestion, and keep your energy stable—something you're definitely going to need when the baby has you up at 3 a.m.

The Power Trio: Protein, Fibre, And Healthy Fats

1. *Protein*
   Protein is your new best mate when it comes to feeling full and maintaining muscle mass. This doesn't mean you need to turn into a bodybuilder. It's simply about choosing foods that help your body repair itself. You've got muscles that need rebuilding—especially if you're hoping to start gentle exercises soon.

What to Eat:

- *Lean meats like chicken or turkey (or if you're veggie, think beans and lentils).*
- *Eggs, which are quick and versatile (boiled, scrambled, poached—whatever you fancy).*
- *Fish (especially oily ones like salmon, packed with omega-3s).*
- *Greek yoghurt (high in protein and can be topped with fruits and seeds).*

Tip: Keep boiled eggs in the fridge as a quick snack. It's not glamorous, but they're protein-packed and can save you from grabbing the biscuits when you're starving.

2. *Fibre*
   Fibre is the unsung hero of the postpartum period. It helps keep you regular—something that becomes oddly important

after birth when your digestive system is in recovery mode. It also keeps you full for longer and stabilises your blood sugar, which means fewer cravings and energy dips.

What to Eat:

- *Whole grains like oats, brown rice, and quinoa. If you're having porridge in the morning, sprinkle in some chia seeds or flaxseeds for an extra fibre boost.*
- *Veggies—especially the green leafy kind. Think spinach, kale, broccoli. If you're not a fan of salads, throw them into a stir-fry or soup.*
- *Fruits with the skin on (apples, pears, and berries are fab for fibre).*

Tip: *Start your day with porridge made with oats, almond milk, and topped with berries and a drizzle of honey. It's quick, filling, and full of fibre.*

3. **Healthy Fats**
   Fat is not the enemy, despite what diet culture might have you believe. You need healthy fats to help balance hormones, keep your brain functioning (hello, baby brain), and give you the energy you need to get through the day.

What to Eat:

- *Avocados (on toast, in salads, or mashed into your eggs—it's hard to go wrong).*
- *Nuts and seeds (almonds, walnuts, and flaxseeds are especially good for boosting omega-3s).*
- *Olive oil and coconut oil for cooking.*
- *Fatty fish like salmon and mackerel.*

Tip: *If you're short on time, throw together a quick snack with avocado mashed onto wholegrain toast, topped with a sprinkle of seeds. It's a powerhouse of healthy fats and fibre in one go.*

Meal Prepping: Your New Best Friend

Look, I get it—meal prepping sounds like something only people with a lot of time on their hands do. But when you're a new mum, it's going to be your secret weapon. Prepping a few meals in advance means you won't be reaching for ready meals or whatever's in the back of the cupboard when you're too exhausted to cook.

Here's a simple meal prep plan that you can knock out in an hour or two (in between feeding the baby, obviously):

1. ***Batch Cook Some Basics:***
   Cook up a big batch of brown rice or quinoa. Keep it in the fridge, and you've got an easy base for meals.
2. ***Roast Some Veggies:***
   Slice up sweet potatoes, carrots, and courgettes, toss them in olive oil, and roast them all at once. These make great add-ons to any meal (or as a quick snack).
3. ***Make a Big Stew or Soup:***
   A hearty vegetable soup or chicken stew can be made in one pot and last you several days. Plus, it's an easy way to get loads of nutrients in one meal.
4. ***Prep Some Snacks:***
   Keep healthy snacks on hand like nuts, fruits, and homemade energy bites (mix oats, peanut butter, and a bit of honey, roll into balls, and freeze). These will be lifesavers when you need something quick.

Tip*: Use freezer bags or containers to portion out meals. Label them with the date so you can grab them in a pinch.*

Hydration: Why It's More Important Than You Think

You know how they say, "Drink more water"? Well, it's not just because you need to stay hydrated—it actually plays a key role in weight loss and recovery. Drinking enough water helps with digestion, keeps your energy up, and stops you from mistaking thirst for hunger (a common mistake).

How Much Water Should You Drink?

The general rule of thumb is 8-10 glasses a day. If you're breastfeeding, you might need a bit more. The easiest way to make sure you're getting enough is to carry a water bottle with you throughout the day. Keep it next to your breastfeeding chair or pram, so you're always reminded to take a sip.

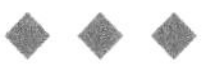

*Common Pitfalls and How
to Avoid Them*

1. ***Skipping Meals***
   When you're juggling a baby and a million other things, it's easy to forget to eat. But skipping meals can backfire, leaving you feeling ravenous later on, which often leads to overeating or grabbing the nearest unhealthy snack.
   Solution*: Try to eat small meals regularly. Even if it's just a piece of toast with peanut butter or a quick smoothie, it's better than nothing.*

2. ***Relying on Sugary Foods for Quick Energy***
   When you're exhausted, it's tempting to reach for something sugary to give you a quick energy boost. The problem is, that energy is short-lived, and you'll crash later.
   Solution*: Instead, opt for snacks that combine protein and fibre, like a handful of almonds with an apple or a small portion of Greek yoghurt with berries.*

3. ***Dieting Too Soon***

The pressure to lose weight after pregnancy is real, but diving into restrictive diets can do more harm than good—especially if your body is still healing.

Solution*: Focus on nourishing your body with balanced meals, and let weight loss come naturally over time. You've got enough on your plate without adding the stress of calorie counting.*

◆ ◆ ◆

Patience, Love, and Food

At the end of the day, your relationship with food postpartum is all about balance. You're fuelling your body, not depriving it. So enjoy your meals, be kind to yourself, and remember that progress takes time. There's no rush to lose the baby weight, and no deadline for getting back to your pre-pregnancy shape. This is about feeling good, rebuilding your energy, and taking care of the amazing body that just gave you the gift of motherhood.

So, go ahead—have that chocolate, but make sure you're also filling your plate with the good stuff that's going to keep you feeling strong and energised for the long haul. You've got this.

CHAPTER 3: GENTLE EXERCISES FOR BODY AND MIND

So, you've made it through the first few weeks of the postpartum haze—congrats! You might be ready to start thinking about getting your body moving again. But before you roll your eyes and throw this book across the room, don't worry: I'm not suggesting you lace up your trainers and start doing star jumps in the living room.

This chapter is all about **gentle**, effective movement. It's not about getting 'fit' in the traditional sense or bouncing back overnight. You're not training for the Olympics (though, to be fair, sometimes just getting through a day with a newborn does feel like a marathon). This is about reconnecting with your body, building up your strength, and healing from the inside out.

◆ ◆ ◆

Weeks 1-6: Rest is Best (But Here's What You Can Do)

First things first: don't rush. Your body has been through a massive physical ordeal, and you need to let it recover. In these first few weeks postpartum, the key is to focus on **rest and recovery**. However, there are a few gentle exercises you can do right now that will help you feel a little more like yourself.

Pelvic Floor Exercises (Kegels)

Yes, we're starting with the pelvic floor—those deep muscles that have worked overtime throughout pregnancy and childbirth. Strengthening your pelvic floor will help with bladder control, support your internal organs, and can even improve your posture. Plus, you can do these exercises anywhere—no one will know!

How To Do Them:

- *Imagine you're trying to stop the flow of urine midstream. Squeeze those muscles, hold for a few seconds, and then release.*
- *Repeat 10 times, and aim to do this a few times throughout the day (you can do it while feeding the baby, lying in bed, or sitting on the sofa).*

Tip: Don't hold your breath! Breathe normally as you contract and release.

◆ ◆ ◆

Walking: The Ultimate Gentle Workout

Even if you're still in your PJs, shuffling around the house, walking is one of the best forms of postpartum exercise. Start slow—just walking around the house or down the street with the pram is a great way to get your body moving again. Walking helps circulation, boosts your mood, and gently engages your muscles without overloading them.

How To Start:

- *In the first few weeks, aim for short walks—around the house, or a brief stroll down the road.*
- *As you feel stronger, you can start increasing the distance, but don't feel pressured to go too far too soon.*

Tip*: If you're struggling to find time, make walking a part of your daily routine. Need to pop to the shops? Take the baby out for a stroll in the pram. Fresh air and gentle movement do wonders for your energy levels.*

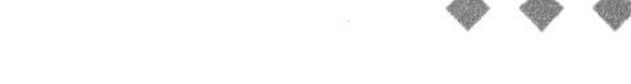

Deep Breathing and Belly Breathing

Your core has been stretched to its limits, and the idea of doing any kind of ab workout might make you cringe. But don't worry —this isn't about crunches or planks. We're starting with **deep breathing** exercises, which help re-engage your core muscles without putting too much strain on them.

How To Do It:

1. *Sit or lie down in a comfortable position.*
2. *Place one hand on your chest and the other on your belly.*
3. *Inhale deeply, letting your belly rise as you breathe in.*
4. *Slowly exhale, drawing your belly button towards your spine.*
5. *Repeat this for 5-10 breaths.*

Tip*: This is also great for relaxing your mind. Try doing this before bed or while the baby is napping to help calm your body and mind.*

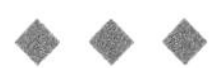

Weeks 6-12: Gentle Strengthening

Once you've got the all-clear from your healthcare provider (usually around the six-week mark), you can start incorporating some gentle strengthening exercises into your routine. Remember, we're not aiming to 'bounce back'—we're building a foundation of strength that will support you in the long run.

Pelvic Tilts

Pelvic tilts are a gentle way to start strengthening your lower back and core without putting too much strain on your body.

How To Do It:

1. *Lie on your back with your knees bent, feet flat on the floor.*
2. *Flatten your lower back against the floor by tilting your pelvis up.*
3. *Hold for a few seconds, then release.*
4. *Repeat 10 times.*

Tip: *Make sure you're breathing throughout the exercise—don't hold your breath!*

Bridge Pose

Bridge pose is a simple exercise that targets your glutes and core, helping to rebuild strength in your lower body.

How To Do It:

1. *Lie on your back with your knees bent and feet flat on the floor.*
2. *Slowly lift your hips up towards the ceiling, squeezing your glutes as you rise.*
3. *Hold for a few seconds at the top, then lower your hips back*

down.

4. *Repeat 10-15 times.*

Tip: *Focus on engaging your core and glutes during this movement. If you feel any discomfort in your lower back, stop and try a gentler exercise.*

Seated Marches

This is a simple exercise that helps engage your core and improve coordination without putting too much strain on your body.

How To Do It:

1. *Sit tall in a chair with your feet flat on the floor.*
2. *Slowly lift one leg at a time, as if you're marching, while keeping your core engaged.*
3. *Alternate legs, lifting each one for a count of three before lowering.*

Tip: *Keep your movements slow and controlled to really engage your core.*

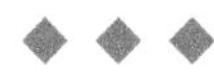

Months 3-6: Gradual Strengthening and Building Confidence

By the three-month mark, you're probably feeling a bit stronger and more confident in your body. Now's the time to start building on that foundation, but we're still going slow and steady. This phase is about increasing your strength and stamina without overwhelming your body.

Bodyweight Exercises

You don't need fancy equipment to start building strength. Using your own bodyweight is one of the most effective ways to rebuild muscle and improve your overall fitness.

Exercises To Try:

- **Squats**: *Stand with your feet hip-width apart. Lower your body as if you're sitting back into a chair, keeping your knees over your toes. Push through your heels to return to standing. Repeat 10-15 times.*
- **Modified Push-Ups**: *Start on your hands and knees. Lower your chest towards the floor while keeping your core engaged. Push back up to the starting position. Repeat 8-10 times.*

Resistance Band Workouts

If you're ready to take things up a notch, resistance bands are a great way to add some gentle resistance without overloading your body. They're cheap, portable, and effective.

Exercises To Try:

- **Bicep Curls with a Resistance Band**: *Stand on the band with both feet and hold the ends in your hands. Curl your arms towards your shoulders, squeezing your biceps as you lift.*
- **Leg Lifts with a Resistance Band**: *Lie on your side with the band looped around your legs, just above your knees. Lift your top leg, squeezing your glutes as you lift, then lower back down.*

Exercise Caution: Diastasis Recti and Overtraining

If you have diastasis recti (a separation of your abdominal muscles), it's important to avoid exercises that can make it worse.

Crunches, sit-ups, and other exercises that put too much strain on your core should be avoided until your muscles have healed.

Safe Alternatives:

- *Stick to exercises like pelvic tilts, bridge pose, and gentle core engagement exercises that don't cause your belly to dome or bulge.*
- *If you're unsure, it's always worth checking in with a physiotherapist who specialises in postpartum recovery.*

And most importantly, listen to your body. If you're feeling overly fatigued or experiencing pain, take it as a sign to rest. Recovery takes time, and each small step is progress.

◆ ◆ ◆

Patience, Progress, and Positivity

Remember, this isn't a race. Postpartum recovery is about taking small, manageable steps that help you rebuild your strength and confidence. Every little bit of movement counts—whether it's a 10-minute walk, a few pelvic tilts, or a full-body stretch while the baby naps. Celebrate every bit of progress, no matter how small.

Your body has done something miraculous, and it deserves to be treated with kindness and care. So keep going, keep moving, and most importantly, keep being kind to yourself. You're doing brilliantly, and you've got this.

CHAPTER 4:
BATTLING FATIGUE:
SLEEP AND ENERGY

If you're a new mum reading this, the words "sleep" and "energy" might seem like a cruel joke. Getting a solid night's sleep feels about as realistic as running a marathon in flip-flops. It's hard to get a decent stretch of shut-eye when you're juggling night feeds, nappy changes, and a baby that seems to know when you've just drifted off.

But here's the good news: while it might not be possible to get your old sleep routine back for a while, there are ways to manage the **chronic tiredness** and **energy slumps** that come with the territory of new motherhood. This chapter is all about how to navigate the fatigue, sneak in rest where you can, and find ways to keep your energy levels up, even when you're running on fumes.

◆ ◆ ◆

The Sleep Struggle Is Real

Let's start by acknowledging one simple fact: **sleep deprivation** is tough. Really tough. It affects everything from your mood to your metabolism, and the lack of sleep can make postpartum recovery feel even more difficult. But here's the thing—you're not going to feel this way forever. Your baby will eventually sleep longer stretches, and so will you. In the meantime, let's focus on how to cope with the sleep you are getting (or, let's be honest, not getting).

Why Sleep is So Important (But Also So Elusive)

When you don't get enough sleep, your body reacts by increasing levels of the hormone **ghrelin**, which makes you feel hungry, and decreasing **leptin**, the hormone that tells you when you're full. This can lead to overeating, especially sugary snacks for quick energy. So, if you've been craving biscuits and cake, that's not just your sweet tooth talking—it's your body's natural response to sleep deprivation.

Not only that, but a lack of sleep affects your emotional wellbeing, making you feel more irritable, anxious, and weepy. So if you've found yourself crying over an ad on telly, don't worry—you're not losing it. You're tired.

Prioritising Rest: Sneaking in Sleep Where You Can

"Sleep when the baby sleeps" is the advice everyone gives, but let's be honest—it's not always that simple. What about when the baby finally naps, but the laundry needs doing, the dishes are piling up, and you haven't showered in three days? Here's a radical idea: sometimes, those things can wait. You don't need to have a perfect house; what you need is to take care of yourself so you can take care of your baby.

◆ ◆ ◆

How to Make Rest a Priority (Even When It Feels Impossible)

1. **Nap Strategically**
    If you can't get long stretches of sleep, aim for short, 20-30 minute naps when the baby sleeps. These 'power naps' can help boost your energy without making you feel groggy. Don't worry about falling into a deep sleep—just resting with your eyes closed can still help recharge you.

2. **Delegate and Ask for Help**
    It's not easy to ask for help, but now is the time to let go of the 'supermum' mentality. Whether it's your partner, a family member, or a friend, don't be afraid to ask someone to watch the baby for an hour while you nap, shower, or just have a moment to yourself. You need it, and you deserve it.

3. **Create a Calm Sleep Environment**
    When you do get the chance to sleep, make sure your environment is as restful as possible. Keep the room cool and dark, use white noise if needed (to drown out any baby monitor noise that might have you on edge), and invest in comfortable bedding. Anything that makes your sleep more restful, even if it's for a short time, is worth it.

4. **Let Go of Guilt**
    It's tempting to use nap times to catch up on housework or respond to texts and emails, but sometimes, it's more important to rest. Remember, it's not selfish to take care of yourself. You'll be a better mum when you're well-rested and not running on empty.

Boosting Energy Without

Burning Out

If a full night's sleep is off the table (which, let's be real, it probably is), the next best thing is figuring out how to manage your energy levels throughout the day. While you might not feel like your old self, there are small adjustments you can make to avoid energy crashes and keep going—without downing cups of coffee all day (although one or two is totally fine!).

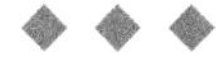

Smart Snacking for Energy

Your energy levels are directly linked to what you eat. If you've been reaching for sugary snacks or caffeine to keep yourself going, you're probably riding the rollercoaster of energy highs and crashes. Instead, focus on snacks that provide **slow-release energy**, keeping you going for longer.

Here are a few easy snack ideas that combine protein and fibre (the dynamic duo for steady energy):

- ***Greek yoghurt with honey and berries****: This is a quick, satisfying snack that gives you protein, fibre, and a touch of sweetness without the sugar crash.*
- ***Hummus with veggie sticks****: Veggies like carrots, cucumbers, and peppers paired with hummus give you fibre, healthy fats, and a satisfying crunch.*
- ***Apple slices with peanut butter****: The apple gives you fibre and natural sugar, while the peanut butter adds protein and healthy fats to keep you feeling full.*

Move (Even When You Don't Feel Like It)

I know, I know—exercise is probably the last thing you want to do when you're exhausted. But here's the thing: gentle movement, like going for a short walk or doing some light stretching, can actually give you a boost of energy. It gets your blood flowing, improves circulation, and helps clear that brain fog that comes from being sleep-deprived.

How To Incorporate Movement:

- *Start small: Even just five minutes of stretching or walking around the house can help.*
- *Take the baby with you: Pop the baby in the pram and head outside for some fresh air. The combination of light exercise and sunshine can do wonders for your mood and energy levels.*

◆ ◆ ◆

Caffeine: Your Friend or Foe?

Caffeine is a lifeline for many new mums, and there's no shame in enjoying your morning cuppa. But too much caffeine can actually backfire, making you jittery and causing energy crashes later on. Plus, if you're breastfeeding, it's best to keep your caffeine intake moderate (around 200-300 mg per day, or roughly one to two cups of coffee).

How To Manage Caffeine (Without Overdoing It):

- ***Enjoy it, but don't rely on it****: Savour your morning coffee, but try not to make it your only source of energy.*
- ***Time it wisely****: Avoid caffeine in the late afternoon or evening, as it can interfere with your sleep later on.*
- ***Hydrate****: Balance your caffeine intake with plenty of water to stay hydrated and avoid that dehydrated sluggish feeling.*

Recharging Mentally: Rest for Your Mind

Physical rest is important, but don't forget about mental rest. Your brain has been on overdrive since the baby arrived, and it needs a break too. Constantly thinking about the baby, the housework, and everything else on your to-do list can leave you feeling mentally drained, even if you've had a bit of sleep.

Ways To Mentally Recharge:

1. ***Take Breaks from Technology***
   Scrolling through social media while you're up for a night feed might seem like a good distraction, but it can actually make you feel more anxious or drained. Try to give your mind a break from the constant barrage of information and notifications. Read a book, listen to calming music, or just sit quietly.

2. ***Mindfulness and Deep Breathing***
   Taking just a few minutes to practise mindfulness or deep breathing can help clear your mind and reduce stress. Focus on your breath, let go of any intrusive thoughts, and give your brain a moment to relax.

3. ***Connect with Friends (But Keep It Light)***
   Social interaction can be energising, but don't feel like you need to keep up with everyone all the time. A short phone call or text exchange with a supportive friend can boost your mood without draining your energy.

Finding Your New Rhythm

At the end of the day, postpartum life is about finding a new rhythm that works for you. It might not be the one you had before the baby arrived, and that's okay. This stage of life is temporary, and your energy levels will improve over time as your baby starts to sleep longer and you regain some control over your schedule.

Until then, the key is to **manage your expectations**, take rest where you can get it, and remember that you're doing an amazing job—no matter how tired you feel.

So, put the kettle on, enjoy that well-deserved cup of tea, and give yourself permission to rest. You've earned it.

CHAPTER 5: REALISTIC FITNESS PLANS FOR BUSY MUMS

By now, you've probably realised that motherhood is an Olympic sport in its own right—minus the medals, but with plenty of "training" (read: multitasking) and "endurance" (read: sleepless nights). Between feedings, nappy changes, and trying to remember if you've had lunch, finding time for fitness might seem like an impossible dream. But the truth is, exercise doesn't have to be a two-hour sweat fest or involve expensive gym memberships. In fact, squeezing in a little movement each day can make a world of difference in your energy levels, mood, and recovery.

This chapter is all about creating **realistic fitness plans** that actually fit into your busy life, without adding any extra pressure. We're focusing on **short, effective workouts** that you can do in between naps, feeds, and maybe even while the baby plays. No fancy equipment required—just you, a bit of space, and a willingness to embrace the chaos.

Why Fitness Post-Baby is Different (and That's Okay)

First things first: let's dispel the myth that postpartum fitness is about getting back to your pre-baby body. It's not. Your body has done something incredible, and it's changed in the process. The goal of postpartum fitness isn't to 'snap back'—it's to **rebuild strength**, **boost energy**, and **support your overall wellbeing**. It's about helping you feel good, not chasing some unrealistic ideal.

Your muscles, joints, and core need time to heal and rebuild, so the exercises you do now should be gentle and supportive, not punishing. You'll also want to pay attention to your pelvic floor and core—these areas take the brunt of pregnancy and delivery, and they need to be strengthened slowly and carefully.

Creating a Fitness Routine That Works for You

The key to making fitness a regular part of your postpartum life is to keep it **simple, flexible, and realistic**. Instead of carving out hours you don't have, try to find pockets of time to fit in short bursts of movement. Even 10 minutes a day can make a difference!

How To Start:

- *Set Small Goals: Instead of aiming to work out for an hour every day, start with something more manageable, like 10 minutes of gentle movement or stretching.*
- *Be Flexible: Some days you'll manage a workout, and other days*

the baby will need all your attention. That's okay—take it one day at a time.

- ***Mix It Up****: Variety is key. Some days you might want to do a bit of strength training, other days a short walk. The goal is to move your body in a way that feels good.*

◆ ◆ ◆

Quick and Effective Workouts for Busy Mums

Here are some easy-to-follow workout routines you can do at home, with minimal equipment and minimal time. You can mix and match these depending on how much time you have and what your body feels up for. These workouts target different areas —core, lower body, and full-body conditioning—to help you build strength gradually.

◆ ◆ ◆

10-Minute Full-Body Workout

No time? No problem. This full-body workout is quick, simple, and can be done anywhere. The goal is to get your blood flowing, work on strength, and give you a boost of energy.

1. ***Squats (1 minute)***
   Stand with your feet shoulder-width apart. Lower down as if sitting back into a chair, keeping your knees in line with your toes. Push through your heels to stand back up. Repeat for one minute.

2. ***Push-Ups (1 minute)***
   Start in a plank position on your knees. Lower your body down towards the floor, keeping your elbows close to your body. Push back up. Modify by keeping your knees on the ground. Repeat for one minute.

3. ***Bridge Pose (1 minute)***
   Lie on your back with your knees bent and feet flat on the floor. Lift your hips towards the ceiling, squeezing your glutes. Lower back down and repeat for one minute.
4. ***Plank Hold (1 minute)***
   Start in a plank position on your forearms or with your hands on the floor. Keep your core engaged and hold for as long as you can, aiming for one minute.
5. ***Lunges (1 minute)***
   Stand with your feet together. Step one foot forward into a lunge, lowering your back knee towards the floor. Push through your front foot to return to standing and alternate legs. Repeat for one minute.
6. ***Rest for 30 seconds***, *then repeat the circuit for another 5 minutes if you can.*

Tip: *If the baby's playing or watching, turn it into a fun game—do squats while holding them or let them join in on the floor for some tummy time while you plank.*

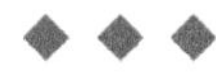

20-Minute Core and Lower Body Strengthening

Your core and lower body are key areas to focus on postpartum, as they take a lot of the strain during pregnancy and childbirth. Strengthening these areas can help with posture, reduce back pain, and improve overall stability.

1. ***Pelvic Tilts (2 minutes)***
   Lie on your back with your knees bent. Tilt your pelvis towards you, pressing your lower back into the floor. Hold for a few seconds, then release. Repeat for two minutes.
2. ***Glute Bridges (2 minutes)***
   Lie on your back with your knees bent. Lift your hips

towards the ceiling, squeezing your glutes. Lower back down and repeat for two minutes.

3. **Side-Lying Leg Lifts (2 minutes on each side)**
   Lie on your side with your legs straight. Lift your top leg towards the ceiling, keeping your core engaged. Lower back down and repeat for two minutes, then switch sides.

4. **Bird-Dog (2 minutes)**
   Get on all fours. Extend your right arm and left leg out in front of you. Hold for a few seconds, then switch sides. This exercise helps with core stability and balance. Repeat for two minutes.

5. **Bodyweight Squats (2 minutes)**
   Stand with your feet shoulder-width apart. Lower into a squat, keeping your weight in your heels and your knees over your toes. Push back up and repeat for two minutes.

6. **Rest for 1 minute**, *then repeat the circuit if time and energy allow.*

Tip: *If the baby's awake, you can place them on a blanket next to you and make it a game of peek-a-boo between exercises!*

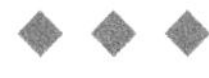

Fitting in Movement: Little and Often

The idea of 'working out' can feel overwhelming, especially when your day is already packed. But what if you stopped thinking of it as a workout and just focused on **moving your body throughout the day**? Here are some simple ways to fit in exercise, without even realising you're doing it:

- **Walk Everywhere**: *Need to pop to the shops? Take the baby in the pram and make it a walking workout. Or simply do laps around the house during nap time.*
- **Stretch While You Wait**: *Waiting for the kettle to boil? Do a few calf raises, shoulder rolls, or side stretches.*
- **Baby-Lifting Workouts**: *Use your baby as a weight! Gently lift*

them up and down while sitting or lying on your back (as long as they're enjoying it, of course).

- **Dance It Out**: *Put on your favourite music and have a mini dance party with the baby. It's a great way to get your heart rate up and have fun at the same time.*

Staying Motivated: It's About Progress, Not Perfection

Staying motivated to exercise when you're exhausted is tough. Some days you'll feel like you can conquer the world, and other days you'll feel like the best you can do is survive. That's normal. The key is to remind yourself that **every little bit of movement counts**—whether it's a five-minute stretch or a 20-minute workout, it all adds up over time.

How to Stay on Track:

1. **Set Realistic Goals**: *Don't aim for perfection. Set small, achievable goals, like working out for 10 minutes a day or taking a walk with the pram. Celebrate every win, no matter how small.*
2. **Track Your Progress**: *Keep a journal or use an app to track your workouts. You'll be amazed at how much progress you've made, even when it feels like nothing's changed.*
3. **Find a Support System**: *Whether it's a friend, partner, or online community, having someone to cheer you on (or commiserate with) can make all the difference.*
4. **Listen to Your Body**: *On the days when you're too tired or just need to rest, that's okay too. Recovery is just as important as exercise, so don't push yourself when you need*

a break.

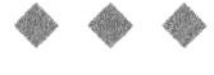

The Key Takeaway: You're Stronger Than You Think

At the end of the day, fitness after baby is about more than just shedding pounds or getting back into old clothes. It's about **rebuilding your strength**, **boosting your energy**, and **feeling good** in your own skin. You've just done something extraordinary—growing and birthing a human—and your body deserves to be treated with kindness and respect.

So keep moving, keep being kind to yourself, and remember: you're stronger than you think. One small step at a time, you're getting stronger, healthier, and more confident every day.

CHAPTER 6: POSTPARTUM MENTAL HEALTH: NURTURING THE MIND AND SPIRIT

While we've talked a lot about your body so far—how it's healing, how to nourish it, and how to move it—we also need to talk about what's going on upstairs. **Your mind**. Because if there's one thing that doesn't get enough attention in the postpartum period, it's mental health. Your emotional wellbeing is just as important as your physical recovery, and it's perfectly normal if you're feeling a bit overwhelmed, emotional, or unlike yourself.

Between the **hormonal changes**, **sleep deprivation**, and the massive life adjustment that comes with a new baby, it's no wonder you're feeling like you're riding a rollercoaster of emotions. Some days, everything will seem fine, and other days, you'll wonder if you're ever going to feel "normal" again. Spoiler alert: You will. But it takes time, patience, and support.

In this chapter, we'll explore **postpartum mental health**, covering everything from the **baby blues** to **postpartum depression**, and how you can take steps to nurture your mind and spirit while navigating this new chapter of life.

The Baby Blues: Why It's Normal to Feel Overwhelmed

You've probably heard of the **baby blues**—that period in the first couple of weeks postpartum when you feel weepy, emotional, and overwhelmed. It's incredibly common, affecting up to 80% of new mums, and usually occurs within the first two weeks after giving birth. It's often triggered by a combination of hormonal shifts, physical exhaustion, and the sudden realisation that your life has changed forever.

What To Expect With The Baby Blues:

- **Tears**: *You might find yourself crying over the smallest things—an advert on telly, a touching song, or even just looking at your baby.*
- **Irritability**: *You may feel easily frustrated, especially when you're tired (and let's face it, you're always tired).*
- **Anxiety**: *It's normal to feel a bit anxious about your new role as a mum, whether it's about breastfeeding, baby's sleep, or just trying to get through the day.*
- **Mood Swings**: *You might feel happy and content one minute, and teary and overwhelmed the next. Again, it's all part of the hormonal changes.*

The good news is that the baby blues typically subside after a couple of weeks. But in the meantime, give yourself grace. It's okay to feel overwhelmed, and it's okay to have a good cry. You've just been through a huge physical and emotional event, and your body is still adjusting.

Postpartum Depression: Knowing When It's More Than the Blues

While the baby blues are common and usually short-lived, **postpartum depression (PPD)** is more serious and can last longer. It's estimated that about 1 in 10 women experience PPD, but many don't seek help because they feel ashamed or afraid of being judged.

Postpartum depression isn't a sign of weakness, and it's not something you've done wrong. It's a medical condition, and it's treatable. If your feelings of sadness, hopelessness, or anxiety last longer than two weeks, or if they're getting worse, it's important to reach out for support.

Signs Of Postpartum Depression:

- ***Persistent feelings of sadness or hopelessness****: If you're feeling down most of the time, or if you're struggling to find joy in things you used to enjoy, it could be a sign of PPD.*
- ***Difficulty bonding with your baby****: Feeling disconnected from your baby, or like you're not able to bond with them, is a common symptom of PPD.*
- ***Irritability or anger****: You might feel easily irritated, or like your patience is wearing thin.*
- ***Sleep disturbances****: Beyond the typical sleep deprivation, you might find that you're unable to sleep even when the baby is sleeping, or you're sleeping too much.*
- ***Thoughts of harming yourself or your baby****: If you're having thoughts of harming yourself or your baby, it's crucial to seek help immediately.*

What To Do If You Think You Have Postpartum Depression:

- ***Speak to your GP or healthcare provider***: Don't hesitate to reach out to your GP, midwife, or health visitor if you think you might be experiencing PPD. They can help you find the right treatment, whether it's therapy, medication, or both.
- ***Join a support group***: Sometimes, just knowing you're not alone can make all the difference. There are support groups for new mums dealing with PPD, both in person and online, where you can share your experiences and connect with others who understand.
- ***Ask for help***: Don't be afraid to lean on your partner, family, or friends during this time. Whether it's asking someone to take the baby for an hour so you can rest or simply talking about how you're feeling, having a support network is vital.

◆ ◆ ◆

Self-Care for Your Mental Wellbeing

We've talked about self-care for your body, but let's talk about **self-care for your mind**. Taking care of your mental health is just as important as physical recovery, and it doesn't have to mean spa days or elaborate routines. It's about finding small moments throughout your day to **recharge**, **reflect**, and **nurture yourself**.

Simple Ways To Practise Self-Care:

1. ***Mindfulness and Meditation***
   Mindfulness is all about being present in the moment, and it can be incredibly calming for an anxious or overwhelmed mind. Even just five minutes of deep breathing or a short meditation can help clear your head and reduce stress.

How to Start:

- *Find a quiet space (even if it's just a few minutes while the baby naps).*

- *Sit comfortably, close your eyes, and focus on your breath. Breathe in slowly, hold for a few seconds, and then exhale.*
- *If your mind starts wandering (which it will), gently bring your attention back to your breath.*

Tip: There are great mindfulness and meditation apps available, like Calm or Headspace, which offer short, guided meditations perfect for busy mums.

◆ ◆ ◆

2. ***Journaling*** *Journaling is a simple, powerful way to process your thoughts and feelings. It can be incredibly helpful for getting all those swirling emotions out of your head and onto paper. You don't need to write pages—just jot down how you're feeling, what's on your mind, or even a few things you're grateful for each day.*

How to Start:

- *Keep a notebook and pen handy, or use a notes app on your phone.*
- *Write for just a few minutes each day. You can start with a simple prompt like, "What am I feeling right now?" or "What's one thing that went well today?"*

Tip: Some mums find it helpful to track their mood alongside their journal entries to see patterns over time. This can be especially useful if you're working with a healthcare provider on managing postpartum depression or anxiety.

◆ ◆ ◆

3. ***Take Time for Yourself (Even Just 10 Minutes)*** *As a new mum, finding time for yourself might seem impossible, but even 10 minutes can make a difference. Whether it's enjoying a cup of tea in peace, taking a warm bath, or simply lying down and closing your eyes, those little pockets*

of time can help recharge your mental batteries.

How to Start:

- *Make it a priority to carve out just a few minutes each day. Ask your partner, a family member, or a friend to watch the baby for a bit while you take a break.*
- *Don't feel guilty for taking time for yourself. You can't pour from an empty cup, and looking after your own wellbeing makes you a better mum.*

Tip*: Schedule these moments of 'me time' just like you would a baby feed or a doctor's appointment. It's easy to put your needs last, but self-care is essential.*

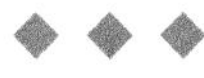

The Power of Support Systems

Having a **support system** can make a world of difference during the postpartum period. Whether it's your partner, family, friends, or fellow mums, surrounding yourself with people who can lift you up is vital for your emotional health. Don't be afraid to lean on others—you're not supposed to do this alone.

Ways To Build And Lean On Your Support System:

1. ***Partner Support****:*
   If you have a partner, talk to them openly about how you're feeling. Let them know what you need, whether it's help with night feeds, taking over a nappy change, or just sitting with you during those tough moments. Communication is key.
2. ***Family and Friends****:*
   Don't be afraid to ask for help, whether it's from your mum, sister, or best friend. Even something as simple as having someone come over to watch the baby while you nap can

make a huge difference. And remember—your loved ones want to help, so let them.

3. ***New Mum Groups:***
   Sometimes, it's helpful to connect with other mums who are going through the same thing. Many communities have new mum groups where you can meet other women, share experiences, and offer support to one another. If meeting in person isn't possible, there are plenty of online forums and groups where you can find support from mums around the world.

When to Seek Professional Help

It's normal to have ups and downs during the postpartum period, but if you're feeling overwhelmed, persistently sad, or unable to cope, it's important to seek professional help. There's no shame in asking for help, and getting support early on can make a huge difference in your recovery.

Signs It's Time To Reach Out:

- *You're feeling down or hopeless most of the time, and it's not improving.*
- *You're having trouble bonding with your baby.*
- *You're experiencing extreme anxiety or panic attacks.*
- *You're struggling to take care of yourself or your baby.*
- *You're having thoughts of harming yourself or your baby.*

What To Do:

- ***Talk to your GP or health visitor:*** *They can help you find the right resources, whether it's therapy, medication, or other forms of support.*

- ***Find a therapist****: Many therapists specialise in postpartum mental health and can help you navigate this challenging time.*
- ***Don't wait****: The sooner you seek help, the sooner you'll start feeling better. Remember, you don't have to go through this alone.*

◆ ◆ ◆

A Journey of Healing

The postpartum period is one of the most transformative times in a woman's life. You're adjusting to a new identity, new responsibilities, and new challenges. Some days will be wonderful, and others will be hard. But no matter what, you're doing an amazing job.

Your mental health matters, and taking care of yourself emotionally is just as important as taking care of your physical health. By practising self-care, seeking support, and giving yourself the space to feel whatever you're feeling, you're setting yourself up for a healthy and strong recovery—both mentally and physically.

CHAPTER 7: REDISCOVERING YOUR IDENTITY AFTER BABY

Becoming a mum is an incredible, life-changing experience, but it's also a journey that can leave you feeling a bit lost. You spend months preparing for the baby's arrival—decorating the nursery, reading parenting books, packing hospital bags—but no one really prepares you for the identity shift that comes with motherhood. Suddenly, you're a mum, and it can feel like the person you used to be has taken a backseat.

This chapter is all about **rediscovering your identity**—because while you are a mum, you're also still **you**. You've just been through a massive transition, and it's perfectly normal to feel like you've lost touch with the things that used to define you. But here's the good news: you don't have to choose between being a mum and being yourself. You can embrace this new chapter of life while still nurturing the person you were before motherhood. It's all about finding **balance**.

◆ ◆ ◆

The "New You" vs. The "Old You"

It's common to feel like you've been split in two—the "new you" who is a mum, and the "old you" who had hobbies, passions, and goals that weren't centred around nappies and night feeds. You might feel pressure to "bounce back" not just physically, but emotionally too. But here's the thing: you don't have to go back to who you were before the baby. In fact, this new version of you is stronger, wiser, and even more capable. The key is finding a way to **blend the old and the new**.

How To Start Reconnecting With Yourself:

1. ***Embrace the Changes***
   It's okay to acknowledge that you've changed. Motherhood is a transformative experience, and it's natural to feel different. Instead of trying to get back to who you were, focus on who you are now and how you want to grow.

2. ***Let Go of Perfectionism***
   *You don't have to be the perfect mum, and you don't have to "bounce back" emotionally or physically. There's no timeline for rediscovering yourself, and it's perfectly okay if it takes time. Be patient with yourself and remember that **progress, not perfection** is the goal.*

3. ***Start Small***
   If you're struggling to remember what used to make you feel like yourself, start small. Think about hobbies or activities you used to love—whether it was reading, painting, going for walks, or meeting up with friends. You don't have to dive in headfirst; even just spending 10 minutes a day doing something that feels like "you" can help you reconnect with yourself.

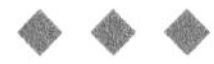

Finding Balance Between
Motherhood and Your Own Needs

One of the hardest parts of motherhood is finding the **balance** between caring for your baby and taking care of yourself. It's easy to feel guilty for wanting time away from your little one, or for missing the independence you had before. But here's the truth: taking time for yourself doesn't make you a bad mum. In fact, it makes you a better one.

Why Self-Care Is Essential:

- ***You're the glue that holds it all together****: If you're running on empty, it's hard to be present for your baby, partner, or even yourself. Taking care of your own needs ensures you have the energy and patience to take care of others.*
- ***It helps prevent burnout****: Motherhood is a marathon, not a sprint. If you don't take breaks to recharge, you risk burnout, which can affect your mental and physical health.*
- ***You deserve it****: You've just gone through a life-altering experience, and you deserve to take time for yourself. Motherhood doesn't mean giving up who you are—it means expanding on it.*

How To Make Time For Yourself:

1. *Ask for Help*
   Don't be afraid to ask your partner, family, or friends for help. Whether it's watching the baby for an hour while you take a bath, or taking over night feeds so you can get a bit more sleep, having a support system can make all the difference. You don't have to do it all on your own.
2. *Schedule "Me Time"*
   It might feel strange to schedule time for yourself, but

sometimes that's the only way to make sure it happens. Set aside 10-15 minutes a day to do something just for you— whether it's reading a book, going for a walk, or even just sitting quietly with a cup of tea.

3. **Set Boundaries**
   It's easy to feel like you have to say "yes" to everything —whether it's visitors, social commitments, or household tasks. But setting boundaries is essential for protecting your time and energy. It's okay to say no to things that don't serve you, and it's okay to prioritise yourself sometimes.

◆ ◆ ◆

Rediscovering Old Passions (And Finding New Ones)

Just because you're a mum doesn't mean you have to give up your hobbies or passions. In fact, finding time to do the things you love is one of the best ways to reconnect with yourself and maintain a sense of identity outside of motherhood.

How To Reintroduce Your Old Passions:

1. **Start Small**
   You don't have to dive back into old hobbies full force. If you loved painting before the baby arrived, start by setting aside 10 minutes a day to doodle or work on a small project. If you loved running, start with short walks or gentle jogs. The key is to reintroduce these activities slowly, without putting too much pressure on yourself.

2. **Blend Your Old Life with Your New Life**
   Sometimes, finding balance is about blending your old life with your new one. If you loved cooking before the baby arrived, try involving your little one in the kitchen as they grow (even if it's just having them watch while you chop

veggies). If you loved going to the gym, consider finding a mum-and-baby fitness class or working out at home with the baby in a sling.

3. **Be Open to New Interests**
Parenthood changes you, and sometimes that means discovering new passions along the way. Maybe you find that you love baby yoga, or maybe you've developed a newfound interest in photography (because let's be honest, you're probably snapping a million baby photos a day). Be open to exploring new hobbies and interests that fit your current lifestyle.

◆ ◆ ◆

Dealing with Mum Guilt

Ah, **mum guilt**. It's something almost every mum experiences at some point, whether it's feeling guilty for taking time for yourself, for not doing enough, or for simply not having all the answers. But here's the thing: you're doing your best, and that's more than enough.

How To Let Go Of Mum Guilt:

1. ***Recognise that it's normal***
Mum guilt is incredibly common, but that doesn't mean it has to control your life. Recognising that these feelings are normal can help you take a step back and put things into perspective.

2. ***Challenge your thoughts***
When you start feeling guilty for taking time for yourself or for not being "perfect," challenge those thoughts. Remind yourself that taking care of yourself makes you a better mum, and that no one—not even the Instagram-perfect mums—has it all together.

3. ***Focus on the positives***
   Instead of dwelling on the things you feel guilty about, focus on the things you're doing well. Are you loving your baby fiercely? Are you keeping them fed, warm, and safe? Those are huge wins, and they're what really matter.

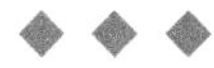

Embracing Your New Identity

At the end of the day, motherhood is about growth, change, and rediscovery. You're not just a mum—you're still you, with all the dreams, goals, and passions you had before. The difference is that now, you've added another layer to your identity: you're stronger, more resilient, and more capable than you've ever been before.

Rediscovering your identity after baby is a journey, and it's okay if it takes time. But with patience, self-care, and a little bit of grace, you'll find a way to balance motherhood with the things that make you feel like yourself.

So go ahead, embrace the changes, nurture the things that make you happy, and remember: you're not just surviving—you're thriving.

CHAPTER 8:
BUSTING THE BOUNCE-BACK MYTH

W e need to have an honest chat about the "bounce-back" culture. You've probably seen it on social media—celebrities and influencers flaunting their "pre-baby bodies" just weeks after giving birth. The flat stomachs, toned legs, and glowing skin, all while juggling a newborn. It's easy to feel a bit disheartened when you're scrolling through Instagram at 3 a.m., feeling anything but glamorous.

But here's the truth: the idea of "bouncing back" is a **myth**—and a harmful one at that. It sets unrealistic expectations for mums who are already dealing with enough pressure. Your body isn't designed to snap back to its pre-baby state immediately (or ever), and it's important to give yourself permission to let go of that goal. This chapter is about embracing the **realities** of postpartum recovery, rejecting the pressure to "bounce back," and celebrating your body for the incredible thing it has just done.

◆ ◆ ◆

Why "Bouncing Back" Is a Myth

Your body has spent nine months growing and nurturing a human being. In that time, it has undergone incredible changes—your uterus expanded, your skin stretched, your hormones fluctuated, and your muscles shifted to make room for your baby. So the idea that your body should "snap back" to its pre-pregnancy state in just a few weeks (or even months) is not only unrealistic, it's unf

air.

Why It Takes Time For Your Body To Heal:

1. ***Your Uterus Needs to Shrink***
   *After giving birth, your uterus doesn't immediately return to its normal size. It can take **six weeks or longer** for your uterus to shrink back down, which means you might still have a bit of a belly for a while—and that's perfectly normal.*

2. ***Hormonal Fluctuations***
   Your hormones are still all over the place after giving birth. Oestrogen and progesterone, which were high during pregnancy, take a nosedive postpartum. This can affect everything from your mood to your metabolism, which means your body is still adjusting.

3. ***Your Muscles Are Healing***
   If you had a vaginal birth, your pelvic floor muscles stretched to allow your baby to come through. And if you had a caesarean section, your abdominal muscles were cut during the surgery. In both cases, it takes time for those muscles to heal and rebuild strength.

4. ***Breastfeeding Doesn't Always Equal Weight Loss***
   While breastfeeding burns extra calories, it doesn't always result in weight loss. Your body may hold onto extra fat

reserves to support milk production, and for some mums, that means the weight doesn't come off as quickly as they'd like.

◆ ◆ ◆

The Pressure to "Snap Back" (And Why It's Harmful)

The pressure to "snap back" comes from all directions—social media, the media in general, and even well-meaning friends and family. But this pressure is harmful because it suggests that your worth is tied to how quickly you can look like you never had a baby in the first place. It reduces your incredible journey of motherhood to a race to fit into old jeans, and that's not only unfair—it's damaging to your self-esteem and mental health.

How To Resist The Pressure:

1. **Curate Your Social Media Feed**
   If scrolling through Instagram leaves you feeling bad about yourself, it's time to hit the "unfollow" button on accounts that promote unrealistic postpartum bodies. Instead, follow accounts that celebrate real, diverse postpartum journeys, and make you feel empowered, not less than.

2. **Challenge the Bounce-Back Narrative**
   When people comment on your body or ask when you're planning to "lose the baby weight," feel free to challenge the narrative. You don't owe anyone an explanation for your body's timeline. Your body is doing exactly what it needs to do—healing and nourishing your baby.

3. **Focus on Function, Not Aesthetics**
   Instead of focusing on getting your pre-baby body back, focus on what your body can do. Can you walk a little further today than you could last week? Can you carry your

baby without pain? These are the victories that matter, not the number on the scale or the size of your jeans.

Celebrating What Your Body Has Done (Instead of Criticising It)

Your body is **amazing**. It has grown and delivered a human being, and that's something to be celebrated, not criticised. When you look at your body postpartum, it's easy to focus on the things that have changed—the stretch marks, the extra weight, the softness around your belly. But instead of criticising those changes, try to celebrate them as a reminder of the incredible thing your body has done.

How To Start Celebrating Your Body:

1. *Shift Your Focus*
   When you look in the mirror, instead of zooming in on the things you wish were different, take a moment to appreciate what your body has done. Those stretch marks? They're proof that your skin stretched to make room for your baby. That soft belly? It protected and nurtured your little one for nine months.

2. *Practice Gratitude*
   Each day, take a moment to express gratitude for something your body has done. It can be as simple as thanking your body for getting you through the day, for nourishing your baby, or for helping you heal.

3. *Speak Kindly to Yourself*
   The way you talk to yourself matters. Instead of criticising yourself, practice speaking kindly to your body. You wouldn't tell a friend that she looks terrible, so why say it to yourself? Treat yourself with the same compassion you

would give to someone else.

Redefining Postpartum Success

Postpartum success shouldn't be defined by how quickly you lose the baby weight or how closely you resemble your pre-pregnancy self. Instead, let's redefine success as feeling **strong, healthy**, and **confident** in your own skin, no matter what that looks like.

Signs Of Postpartum Success (That Have Nothing To Do With Weight):

1. ***You're Feeling Stronger***
   Success isn't about a number on a scale—it's about feeling stronger and more capable each day. Whether that means walking a little further, lifting your baby without pain, or feeling more energised, those are the milestones that matter.

2. ***You're Rebuilding Confidence***
   Rebuilding your confidence postpartum is a process, but every step you take towards feeling good in your own skin is a victory. Whether it's getting dressed in something that makes you feel good or just looking in the mirror and feeling proud of what you've accomplished, that's a win.

3. ***You're Prioritising Your Mental and Physical Health***
   Success isn't just about physical health—it's about mental health too. If you're making time to care for your emotional wellbeing, whether through self-care, therapy, or simply asking for help when you need it, that's a huge success.

Embracing Your Post-Baby Body

At the end of the day, the idea of "bouncing back" is a myth because there's no going back to the way things were. Your body has changed, and that's a beautiful thing. Instead of focusing on getting back to your pre-baby body, embrace the **new version** of yourself—the version that's stronger, more resilient, and more capable than ever.

Your body tells the story of your journey into motherhood, and that's something to be proud of. So let go of the pressure to bounce back, and instead focus on moving forward—one step at a time, with kindness, patience, and gratitude for all that your body has done and will continue to do.

You've got this, mama. And you're already amazing, just as you are.

CHAPTER 9: ADVANCED POSTPARTUM FITNESS: BUILDING STRENGTH WHEN YOU'RE READY

By now, you've had some time to settle into motherhood, and you might be feeling ready to take your fitness journey to the next level. The early postpartum days were all about gentle recovery, reconnecting with your body, and adjusting to life with a baby. Now, whether it's been three months or a year, you might feel a bit stronger, more confident, and ready to incorporate more challenging movements into your routine. This chapter is all about advanced postpartum fitness—but don't worry, we're not talking about punishing workouts or unattainable goals. We're talking about building strength, stamina, and feeling empowered in your body again.

The key is to listen to your body. Postpartum fitness isn't a race, and everyone's timeline looks different. Some mums feel ready to ramp up their workouts after a few months, while others need more time. Both are perfectly okay. This chapter is about meeting you where you are and helping you progress in a way that feels **sustainable** and **nurturing**.

When You Know You're Ready for More

So, how do you know if you're ready to start stepping up your fitness routine? Here are a few signs that your body might be ready for more advanced exercises:

1. ***You're Feeling Stronger***
   You're no longer feeling fatigued by the basics. The gentle exercises you started with—like pelvic tilts, walking, and light stretching—are starting to feel easier, and you feel ready for more.

2. ***Your Core and Pelvic Floor Are More Stable***
   You're able to engage your core muscles without feeling discomfort or noticing doming (a bulge in the middle of your abdomen, which could indicate diastasis recti). Your pelvic floor feels stronger, and you're not experiencing leaks or discomfort during everyday activities.

3. ***You Have More Energy***
   Instead of feeling drained after a short workout, you're finding that exercise is giving you energy and boosting your mood.

4. ***You've Been Cleared by Your Healthcare Provider***
   If you've had a check-up with your GP, midwife, or physiotherapist, and they've given you the all-clear to start incorporating more advanced exercises, then you're good to go!

Strength Training for Busy Mums

One of the most effective ways to build muscle and improve overall fitness is through **strength training**. This doesn't mean you need to lift heavy weights or spend hours in the gym—simple bodyweight exercises, resistance bands, or light weights can help you build strength gradually. Strength training not only helps you tone your body, but it also **boosts your metabolism**, improves posture, and gives you more stamina to keep up with your little one.

Why Strength Training Is Important Postpartum:

1. ***Rebuilds Muscle***: *During pregnancy, your muscles, especially in your core and lower body, stretched and weakened. Strength training helps you rebuild that muscle in a way that supports your body's recovery.*
2. ***Improves Posture***: *Carrying a baby, breastfeeding, and pushing a pram can take a toll on your posture, leading to back and neck pain. Strengthening your back, shoulders, and core helps improve your posture and reduces pain.*
3. ***Boosts Energy***: *Strength training increases your energy levels by improving circulation, releasing endorphins, and building stamina.*
4. ***Supports Weight Loss***: *While weight loss isn't the primary goal of postpartum fitness, strength training can help support healthy weight loss by increasing your lean muscle mass, which burns more calories at rest.*

Advanced Strength Training

Exercises to Try

Here are a few simple strength training exercises you can incorporate into your routine. These exercises target key areas like your core, glutes, arms, and legs, helping you build overall strength while supporting your postpartum recovery.

1. Squats with a Resistance Band

- **Targets**: *Glutes, hamstrings, quads*
- **How to Do It**: *Place a resistance band just above your knees. Stand with your feet hip-width apart. Lower your body into a squat position, keeping your knees in line with your toes. Push through your heels to return to standing. Repeat 10-15 times.*
- **Why It's Great**: *Squats strengthen your glutes and legs, which are essential for lifting, carrying, and chasing after your little one.*

2. Modified Push-Ups

- **Targets**: *Chest, shoulders, arms, core*
- **How to Do It**: *Start in a kneeling plank position, with your hands slightly wider than shoulder-width apart. Lower your chest towards the floor, keeping your elbows close to your body. Push back up to the starting position. Repeat 10-12 times.*
- **Why It's Great**: *Push-ups strengthen your upper body and core, which are crucial for lifting your baby and improving posture.*

3. Glute Bridge with March

- **Targets**: *Glutes, hamstrings, core*
- **How to Do It**: *Lie on your back with your knees bent and feet flat on the floor. Lift your hips towards the ceiling, squeezing your glutes. Once in the bridge position, lift one foot off the floor, keeping your knee bent, and march it towards your chest. Lower the foot back down and repeat on the other side. Continue alternating for 10-12 reps per leg.*
- **Why It's Great**: *This exercise strengthens your glutes and core while also engaging your hip flexors for added stability.*

4. Plank to Side Plank

- **Targets**: Core, obliques, shoulders
- **How to Do It**: Start in a plank position, with your hands directly under your shoulders. Shift your weight onto one hand, and rotate your body to the side, lifting your other arm towards the ceiling. Hold the side plank for a few seconds, then return to the centre and repeat on the other side. Repeat 8-10 times.
- **Why It's Great**: This move strengthens your entire core, including your obliques, which helps with overall core stability.

◆ ◆ ◆

Incorporating Cardio: Low-Impact and Effective

While strength training is key for building muscle, **cardio** is great for improving your heart health, boosting your endurance, and burning calories. The good news is that you don't need to spend hours on a treadmill to get the benefits of cardio. There are plenty of low-impact cardio options that are effective and easy on your joints—perfect for postpartum recovery.

Low-Impact Cardio Ideas:

1. **Walking with the Pram**
   Walking is one of the best forms of postpartum exercise. It's gentle on your body, easy to fit into your day, and can be done with your baby in tow. Try adding in some intervals to increase the intensity—walk briskly for 2 minutes, then slow down for 2 minutes, and repeat for 20-30 minutes.
2. **Swimming**
   Swimming is a full-body workout that's easy on your joints. Whether you're doing gentle laps or participating in a water aerobics class, swimming helps build cardiovascular

endurance without putting strain on your body.

3. **Dancing**

   Put on your favourite playlist and have a mini dance party in the living room. It's a fun way to get your heart rate up, and your baby will love watching you move!

◆ ◆ ◆

Fitting Fitness into Your Day

As a busy mum, finding time to work out can feel like a challenge, but with a little creativity, you can fit fitness into your day without feeling overwhelmed. Here are a few ways to make it happen:

1. **Break It Up**

   You don't need to block out an hour to work out. Instead, try breaking your workout into 10-15 minute chunks throughout the day. Do a quick set of squats in the morning, some push-ups in the afternoon, and a short walk in the evening. It all adds up!

2. **Multitask with Baby**

   If your baby is awake, include them in your workout! You can do squats while holding your baby, use them as added resistance for glute bridges, or go for a brisk walk with the pram.

3. **Set a Schedule**

   If you can, try to schedule your workouts just like you would any other appointment. This helps make it a priority and keeps you accountable. Even if it's just a quick 20-minute session, having it scheduled can help ensure it happens.

◆ ◆ ◆

Exercise Caution: Listening to Your Body

As you start incorporating more advanced exercises, it's important to continue **listening to your body**. Pushing yourself too hard too soon can lead to injury or burnout, so take it slow and pay attention to how your body feels.

What To Watch Out For:

- ***Pain or Discomfort****: If you feel pain (especially in your pelvic area, lower back, or abdomen), stop the exercise and rest. Pain is your body's way of telling you that something isn't right.*
- ***Diastasis Recti****: If you notice doming or bulging in your abdomen during core exercises, it could be a sign that your abdominal muscles haven't fully healed. In this case, avoid exercises like planks or crunches and focus on more gentle core work.*
- ***Excessive Fatigue****: If you're feeling overly exhausted after a workout, it might be a sign that you need to scale back. Recovery is just as important as exercise, especially during postpartum recovery. If you're feeling drained after a workout rather than energised, it's a sign to slow down and give your body the rest it needs.*

◆ ◆ ◆

Staying Motivated as a Busy Mum

Motivation can come and go, especially when you're juggling the demands of motherhood, but staying consistent with your fitness routine is all about finding ways to keep it enjoyable and sustainable. Here are some tips to help you stay motivated:

1. Set Small, Achievable Goals

Rather than aiming for big, long-term goals (like losing a certain amount of weight or running a marathon), focus on smaller, more manageable goals. This could be something like increasing your strength, completing a certain number of workouts each week, or being able to lift your baby with more ease.

2. Celebrate Every Victory

Whether you've managed to fit in a 15-minute workout or you're noticing more energy throughout the day, celebrate your wins. Every bit of progress counts, and acknowledging your achievements can help keep you motivated.

3. Find a Workout Buddy

Having someone to work out with can make the experience more fun and hold you accountable. Whether it's your partner, a friend, or another mum, having a workout buddy can provide support and encouragement.

4. Make it Fun

If you dread your workouts, you're less likely to stick with them. Find exercises that you actually enjoy, whether it's dancing, hiking, swimming, or even playing with your baby. The more fun you have, the more likely you are to keep going.

◆ ◆ ◆

Embrace the Process

At the end of the day, advanced postpartum fitness is about **progress, not perfection**. It's about giving your body the strength and care it needs while honouring the incredible journey it's been on. There will be days when you feel strong and ready to tackle a tough workout, and there will be days when you need rest—and that's okay.

The key is to embrace the process, celebrate your body for what it can do, and continue moving forward at a pace that works for you. Whether you're lifting weights, doing yoga, or going for a walk, every step you take towards rebuilding your strength is a victory worth celebrating.

Remember: You're stronger than you think, and your body is capable of amazing things. So keep going, keep moving, and most importantly, keep being kind to yourself. You've got this.

CHAPTER 10: HOW TO BUILD LONG-TERM SUSTAINABLE HABITS

You've made it through the whirlwind of the early postpartum days. You've started to reconnect with your body, your mind, and maybe even found a little time to remember who you are outside of nappies and night feeds. So, what now? How do you ensure that all the effort you've put into your recovery sticks? That's where building long-term sustainable habits comes in.

Let's be real: motherhood is unpredictable. One minute you're rocking the baby to sleep, the next you're wearing their dinner, and somewhere in between you're supposed to look after yourself too. Sustainable habits are about finding a **balance** that works for you and can be maintained even when life feels a bit chaotic. It's about setting yourself up for success—not perfection. This chapter will help you understand how to **create routines** and **build habits** that fit into your life, so you can continue to thrive without feeling overwhelmed or guilty.

Why Sustainable Habits Matter

Let's start with why habits matter in the first place. When you're in the trenches of motherhood, it's easy to put yourself at the bottom of the priority list. You think, "I'll start exercising again when the baby's older," or, "I'll eat healthier once things calm down." But here's the thing: waiting for the "perfect" time to focus on yourself isn't realistic. Life is busy, and there's always going to be something demanding your attention. Building sustainable habits allows you to **take care of yourself** consistently, even when life throws you a curveball (or a toddler tantrum).

Sustainable habits are small, achievable steps that, over time, make a big impact. It's about creating a foundation of wellness —both mental and physical—that supports you in your everyday life.

Start Small and Be Realistic

The biggest mistake we make when trying to build new habits is **setting the bar too high**. We think we need to overhaul our entire life in one go—start exercising five days a week, cut out sugar, meditate daily, and sleep eight hours every night. Sounds lovely, right? But in reality, when you're already stretched thin, this kind of all-or-nothing approach is a recipe for burnout.

The key to long-term success is starting **small**. Instead of aiming for perfection, aim for progress. Choose one or two habits that feel manageable and build from there.

Examples Of Small Habits To Start With:

1. ***Five Minutes of Movement:*** *On days when you can't fit in a full workout, commit to five minutes of gentle movement. Whether it's stretching, doing a few squats, or taking a brisk walk, it all adds up.*

2. ***Drink More Water****: Start by adding one extra glass of water to your day. Hydration is a simple yet effective way to boost your energy and support your overall health.*

3. ***Daily Gratitude****: Before bed, jot down one thing you're grateful for each day. This habit helps shift your focus towards the positive and can have a big impact on your mental wellbeing.*

◆ ◆ ◆

Habit Stacking: Building New Routines into Existing Ones

If you're struggling to find time for new habits, one of the best ways to integrate them into your life is through something called **habit stacking**. The idea is simple: you take an existing habit—something you already do regularly—and "stack" a new habit on top of it. By linking the new habit with something you're already doing, it becomes easier to remember and eventually becomes part of your routine.

Examples Of Habit Stacking:

- ***While the kettle's boiling****: Do some gentle stretches or deep breathing exercises.*
- ***During nappy changes****: Engage your pelvic floor by doing a few Kegels.*
- ***Brushing your teeth****: Use this time to practice gratitude—think about one thing you're thankful for that day.*

By pairing your new habits with things you're already doing, you make them feel less like an added task and more like a natural part of your day.

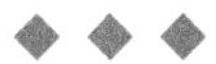

The Importance of Flexibility and Self-Compassion

We've all been there: you set a goal, you're doing great for a few days, and then—bam! Life happens. The baby has a bad night, you're exhausted, and suddenly, the healthy habits you've worked so hard to build feel impossible to maintain. This is where **flexibility** and **self-compassion** come into play.

It's important to understand that building sustainable habits doesn't mean being perfect all the time. It's about being adaptable and **forgiving yourself** when things don't go to plan. Some days, you might nail your workout, drink all your water, and feel on top of the world. Other days, it's an achievement just to get through without crying over spilled milk (literally or figuratively).

How To Stay Flexible:

- *Give yourself permission to adjust: If you're too tired to do your usual workout, do something lighter instead. The important thing is that you're still moving your body, even if it's at a slower pace.*
- *Let go of guilt: If you miss a day (or a few days), don't beat yourself up. Life happens. Instead of focusing on what you didn't do, focus on what you can do next.*
- *Celebrate small wins: Every bit of progress counts, no matter how small. Did you drink more water today? Amazing. Did you manage a 10-minute walk? Brilliant. Celebrate those wins.*

Accountability: Keeping Yourself on Track

Let's be honest: sticking to new habits can be tricky when

you're juggling the demands of motherhood. That's why finding ways to hold yourself accountable can make a big difference. Accountability doesn't mean punishing yourself for not sticking to a plan—it's about setting up a system that keeps you motivated and on track, even on the tough days.

Ways To Stay Accountable:

1. **Buddy Up**: Having someone to share your progress with can make a world of difference. Whether it's a friend, partner, or even an online community of other mums, having someone to check in with can help you stay motivated.
2. **Track Your Progress**: Use a habit tracker, journal, or even an app to keep track of your habits. Seeing your progress visually can be a great motivator and help you stay consistent.
3. **Reward Yourself**: Celebrate your successes! Treat yourself to something special when you hit a milestone —whether it's a relaxing bath, a new book, or just a quiet moment to yourself. Rewards can help reinforce positive behaviour and keep you motivated.

◆ ◆ ◆

Building a Balanced Routine

As you work towards building sustainable habits, it's important to remember that balance is key. Your goal shouldn't be to do everything all at once. Instead, focus on creating a routine that feels balanced and supports your physical and mental wellbeing.

◆ ◆ ◆

What Does a Balanced

Routine Look Like?

- **Movement**: *Aim for a little bit of movement every day, whether it's a full workout, a walk, or some gentle stretching.*
- **Rest**: *Make time for rest and relaxation. Sleep when you can, and give yourself permission to take breaks.*
- **Nutrition**: *Focus on nourishing your body with balanced, healthy meals. And don't forget to enjoy the occasional treat without guilt.*
- **Mental Wellbeing**: *Make self-care a priority, whether it's through mindfulness, journaling, or simply taking a few minutes to breathe.*

◆ ◆ ◆

The Long Game: Embracing Progress Over Perfection

At the end of the day, building long-term sustainable habits is about **progress**, not perfection. There will be ups and downs, good days and bad days, but what matters most is that you keep going. Even when life gets busy, even when you're exhausted, even when things don't go to plan—every small step you take towards taking care of yourself is a win.

Remember, you're not just building habits for a short-term goal; you're creating a lifestyle that supports your wellbeing in the long run. So be kind to yourself, stay flexible, and most importantly, keep going. You've got this.

CONCLUSION: YOU'VE GOT THIS, MUM

So, here we are at the end of the book—but really, this is just the beginning of your journey. Whether you're weeks, months, or even years postpartum, what matters most is that you've made the decision to take care of yourself, both physically and mentally. And that is no small feat, especially when you're juggling the demands of motherhood, family, and everything else life throws at you.

Throughout these pages, we've covered everything from gentle postpartum exercises to strengthening your mental health, to building long-term habits that actually stick. It's been a journey of self-care, self-discovery, and finding the balance between being a mum and being you.

But let's be honest: motherhood is messy, unpredictable, and, at times, completely overwhelming. There will be days when everything goes to plan, and days when it feels like everything is falling apart. And that's okay. **Perfection isn't the goal here**. Progress is.

What you've learned through this process is how to listen to your body, how to move it in ways that make you feel good, and how to nourish it without guilt. You've learned that your mental health is just as important as your physical health, and that asking for help or taking time for yourself isn't selfish—it's essential.

A New Chapter, A New You

As you move forward, remember that this isn't about "getting back" to the person you were before the baby. You're evolving, growing, and becoming someone new—someone stronger, more resilient, and more capable than ever before. You've gone through an incredible transformation, and that deserves to be celebrated.

Motherhood has added a new layer to who you are, but it doesn't define everything about you. You're still allowed to have dreams, passions, and goals that go beyond the nappy bag. You're allowed to take up space, focus on your health, and pursue your happiness —because when you take care of yourself, you're also taking care of your family. A healthier, happier you means a healthier, happier household.

Embrace the Journey

The road ahead isn't always going to be smooth, but you've already proven that you're more than capable of handling whatever life throws at you. You've got the tools now—whether it's taking a deep breath in the middle of a chaotic day, doing a few Wall Pilates moves to strengthen your core, or simply sitting down with a cup of tea and allowing yourself to rest.

Building a life that supports your physical and mental wellbeing is a journey, not a destination. And along the way, there will be moments of triumph, moments of frustration, and everything in between. But no matter what, remember this: **you've got this.**

Keep Going, Keep Growing

So, what's next? That's up to you. Maybe you'll revisit some of the exercises in this book, or maybe you'll try something new. Maybe you'll focus on building habits that help you feel more balanced, or maybe you'll simply take it one day at a time, adjusting as you go.

Whatever path you choose, know that you're not alone. There are countless other mums walking alongside you, facing similar challenges and celebrating similar wins. You've joined a community of women who are navigating this wild, wonderful journey of motherhood, and you're doing brilliantly.

So, go ahead—keep going, keep growing, and keep being the incredible mum (and person) you are. You've got the strength, the resilience, and the grace to handle whatever comes next.

And don't forget: you've already done the hardest thing. The rest is just building on the amazing foundation you've already created.

You've got this, Mum.

ABOUT THE AUTHOR

Lauren Nikora

Lauren Nikora is a devoted mum to two daughters and has dedicated her life to parenting, mental health, and long-life fitness. With a deep passion for supporting other mums in finding balance, she shares her journey of navigating motherhood while prioritising health and wellbeing. Her work focuses on empowering women to embrace sustainable fitness routines and mental wellness strategies that support them not just in the early years, but throughout their lives.